DOES DRINKING MORE WATER HELP YOU LOSE WEIGHT

WEIGHT LOOSING STRATEGIES FOR ALL

KATE .P

Contents

CHAPTER ONE

INTRODUCTION

The idea that increasing your water intake will help you lose weight has received a lot of attention lately. Increased water consumption, according to proponents, can increase metabolism, decrease appetite, and aid in calorie burning. But there are many different factors at play in the intricate interaction between drinking water and losing weight.

This talk will look at the possible advantages of increasing water consumption for managing weight, analyze the data from science to back up this idea, and offer helpful advice on how to lead a healthy lifestyle that includes enough hydration.

Come discuss this topic with us: Does drinking more water aid in weight loss?

The connection between drinking water and losing weight

Researchers, medical experts, and the general public have all expressed a great deal of interest in and discussion on the connection between drinking water and losing weight. Although some research indicates that drinking more water may help with weight loss, the data is conflicting, and it's unclear what mechanisms underlie this relationship.

Water consumption may have an impact on weight loss in the following ways:

Water consumption before to meals has been shown to suppress hunger and limit calorie intake, which in turn lowers total energy consumption. According to certain research, drinking water before to meals might enhance feelings of fullness, potentially leading to a reduction in the number of calories ingested during the meal.

Enhanced Metabolic Rate: Research indicates that consuming cold water could momentarily increase metabolism since it forces the body to use energy to bring the water's temperature up to body temperature. Over time, this rise in metabolic rate may help people burn more calories and lose weight, though the impact will probably be small.

water and Fat Metabolism: Optimal metabolic function, which includes fat metabolism, depends on adequate water. Dehydration can interfere with metabolic functions and make it more difficult for the body to burn fat for energy. People can support their body's capacity to digest fat and encourage weight loss by drinking enough water.

Water Retention and Bloating: On the other hand, bloating and water retention can result from dehydration or from consuming insufficient fluids, which might momentarily raise body weight. Staying hydrated can help people feel less bloated and retain less water, which will temporarily lower their scale weight.

Effect of Substitution: Drinking water instead of high-calorie drinks like sugar-filled sodas, juices, or alcoholic beverages can help lower total caloric intake and aid in weight loss. Drinking water instead of caloric drinks allows people to cut back on their daily energy intake without experiencing any deprivation.

It's crucial to remember that while these mechanisms point to possible advantages of drinking more water for weight loss, the impact of water on weight management is probably influenced by a number of variables, such as individual differences, dietary patterns, levels of physical activity, and general lifestyle choices.

Furthermore, although some research has shown a link between consuming more water and losing weight or consuming less calories, causality has not been proven. To better understand the mechanisms underlying water consumption's significance in weight loss, more research is required.

Although consuming more water can help with weight management in some ways, such as by reducing hunger and promoting hydration, it is not a miracle cure for weight loss. For overall health and well-being, drinking enough water is essential as part of a balanced diet and healthy lifestyle; however, when attempting to lose weight, it should be taken into account in addition to other elements like food selections, exercise, and behavior modification techniques.

Mechanisms of Water Consumption in Loss of Weight

Water consumption may affect weight reduction through a variety of complex methods that may include many physiological processes. Although the precise processes are still unclear, a number of theories have been put out to explain how consuming more water may help people lose weight:

Appetite Suppression: Having a glass of water prior to eating may assist increase feelings of fullness and curb hunger, which may result in consuming fewer calories throughout meals.

Water can physically fill the stomach and reduce appetite because it has no calories and occupies space in the stomach. As a result, people may consume less calories overall, which may aid in weight loss.

Enhanced Satiety: Water may affect satiety signals in the brain in addition to filling the stomach. According to certain research, drinking water may activate stomach and intestinal receptors, sending messages to the brain that enhance sensations of contentment and fullness. This may result in less food being consumed, which will aid in weight loss.

Calorie Replacement: You can cut your overall calorie intake by substituting water for calorie-containing drinks such sugary sodas, juices, or alcoholic beverages. Individuals can reduce their daily energy consumption without experiencing deprivation by switching water for high-calorie beverages, potentially leading to weight loss in the long run.

Elevated Metabolic Rate: Research indicates that consuming cold water could momentarily elevate metabolic rate. Thermogenesis is the process by which the body uses energy to raise the temperature of cold water to body temperature. Even if the effect is brief and mild, it might encourage increased calorie burning and help with weight loss attempts.

water and Fat Metabolism: Optimal metabolic function, which includes fat metabolism, depends on adequate water. Dehydration can interfere with metabolic functions and make it more difficult for the body to burn fat for energy. People can support their body's capacity to digest fat and encourage weight loss by drinking enough water.

Decrease in Water Retention: Ironically, drinking enough water will help prevent bloating and water retention, which can lead to a brief rise in body weight. People who drink enough water may be able to help the body maintain its fluid equilibrium, which could temporarily lower their scale weight.

Although these mechanisms point to the advantages of drinking more water for weight loss, it's crucial to remember that each person will react differently, and water by itself is unlikely to result in noticeable weight loss without concomitant dietary and lifestyle changes.

Overall, increasing water consumption may help with weight management in certain situations, but it should only be seen as one component of a holistic strategy for a healthy diet and lifestyle that also includes behavior modification techniques, regular exercise, and balanced nutrition for long-term weight management and general wellbeing.

Hydration and Regulating Appetite

Hydration affects sensations of hunger and fullness and is essential for controlling appetite.

Here's how hunger regulation is affected by hydration:

Hunger vs. Thirst: Sometimes people mistakenly believe they are hungry when they are truly thirsty, which causes them to eat. Drinking enough water will help you distinguish between hunger and thirst signals, which lowers the chance that you'll consume extra calories.

Increased Satiety: Consuming water prior to meals might make you feel more satisfied and full, which will make you eat fewer calories throughout meals. Water occupies stomach space, which can physically fill the stomach and reduce hunger. As a result, people may consume less calories overall, aiding in weight management.

Appetite Suppression: Studies indicate that water consumption may help reduce appetite by influencing hormones and brain circuits that control hunger. Water consumption, for instance, may activate stomach and intestinal receptors, sending messages to the brain that enhance sensations of fullness and satisfaction.

Calorie-Free Hydration: Drinking mostly water to stay hydrated guarantees that you are not consuming any calories from fluids. Water does not add calories to the diet, unlike sugary drinks and snacks, so it's a great option for relieving thirst and remaining hydrated without increasing calorie consumption.

Post-Meal Hydration: Sipping water after a meal can also facilitate better digestion and satiety.

After a meal, drinking water can aid in the digestion and absorption of nutrients, promote fullness and pleasure, and possibly lessen the need for high-calorie snacks or other foods.

Hydration and Metabolism: Enough water is needed to support healthy metabolic processes, such as the breakdown of proteins, lipids, and carbohydrates. Dehydration may interfere with metabolic functions and have an impact on appetite control. People can impact appetite management and support their body's metabolic processes by maintaining adequate hydration.

All things considered, sustaining proper hydration is critical for bolstering appetite regulation, encouraging fullness, and supporting weight management initiatives. Fruits, vegetables, and herbal teas are examples of foods and drinks high in water content that can be included in the diet to help regulate appetite and stay hydrated throughout the day.

Weight Variations and Water Retention

Water retention may be a factor in both transient increases in scale weight and variations in body weight. This is how variations in weight can be impacted by water retention:

Consumption of Sodium: Consuming too much sodium might cause water retention. An electrolyte that aids in controlling the body's fluid balance is sodium. Excessive sodium intake, which is frequently present in packaged and processed meals, can make the body retain water, which can result in brief weight rises.

Hormonal Changes: Water retention may be impacted by hormonal changes, especially in women throughout the menstrual cycle. Elevations in scale weight may be a result of bloating and water retention brought on by changes in estrogen and progesterone levels, which can also impact fluid balance.

Intake of Carbohydrates: The body stores carbohydrates as glycogen in addition to water. Water retention results from the binding of newly restored glycogen reserves to water molecules. Meals heavy in carbohydrates or intervals of elevated carbohydrate consumption may cause a transient rise in water weight.

Dehydration: Ironically, losing too much fluids might cause the body to retain water. Fluid retention is the result of the body holding onto water as a defense mechanism when it is dehydrated. This may happen as a result of dehydration, profuse perspiration, or specific medical disorders.

Inflammation: The body's inflammatory reaction, whether brought on by an accident, an infection, or long-term problems, can cause fluid retention. Increased blood artery permeability from inflammatory cytokines can lead to fluid leakage into tissues, which can result in swelling and water retention.

Medication: Fluid retention is a side effect of several medications, including corticosteroids, nonsteroidal anti-inflammatory drugs (NSAIDs), and several antidepressants. Due to water retention, people taking these drugs may temporarily gain more weight than usual.

Dietary Factors: A person's food preferences or eating habits may have an impact on water retention. While diets abundant in fruits, vegetables, and whole grains may have a diuretic impact and assist prevent water retention, diets high in processed foods, sodium, and refined carbs may encourage fluid retention.

It's crucial to remember that weight changes and water retention are frequently transient and might occur every day. They might not accurately represent shifts in body fat percentage or general health. For the majority of people, variations in scale weight brought on by water retention are typical and unproblematic.

People can concentrate on staying hydrated, cutting back on sodium, eating a balanced diet full of whole foods, controlling their stress levels, and getting regular exercise to reduce water retention and improve general well-being. It is best to seek advice and evaluation from a healthcare provider if substantial water retention continues or is accompanied by additional symptoms.

Techniques to Increase Water Consumption

Drinking more water is crucial for sustaining hydration and promoting general health. The following are some practical tips to encourage you to sip water more frequently during the day:

Establish a Daily Objective: To begin, decide how much water you will consume each day. Although it's generally advised to consume eight 8-ounce glasses of water or more each day, each person's requirements may differ depending on their age, weight, degree of activity, and environment.

Use a Water Bottle: Whether you're at home, at work, or on the run, keep a reusable water bottle with you at all times. Having access to water at all times facilitates staying hydrated and encourages regular drinking.

Monitor Your Intake: Use a journal, an app, or just scratching off the amount of water you consume each day on a calendar to keep track of how much you consume. You can make sure you're meeting your hydration goals and maintain accountability by keeping an eye on your intake.

Infuse with Flavor: Infuse your water with fruits, herbs, or vegetables to give it a naturally occurring flavor. For added flavor and enjoyment, try adding slices of lemon, lime, cucumber, or berries to your water.

Set Reminders: Remind yourself to stay hydrated throughout the day by setting alarms, using calendar notifications, or using applications on your smartphone. Establish reminders for yourself, for example, every hour or right before each meal.

Drink Before Meals: Establish the practice of having a glass of water prior to every meal. This keeps you hydrated, but it can also help you eat less calories by encouraging feelings of fullness and decreasing the chance that you will overeat.

Sip Throughout the Day: Try to sip water continuously throughout the day as opposed to attempting to down enormous volumes of it all at once. When you're feeling thirsty, or when you take regular breaks from your everyday activities, take little sips.

CHAPTER TWO

Swap Sugary Drinks: Water should be used in place of sugary drinks including soda, sweetened tea, and sports drinks. This encourages improved hydration in addition to reducing calories and added sugar intake.

Establish Hydration objectives: Include water-drinking challenges in your daily routine to push yourself to reach your hydration objectives. For instance, you may set a goal to consume a specific amount of water bottles by the end of the day or monitor your advancement toward a weekly hydration objective.

Make Water Accessible: Throughout your house and office, keep water bottles or glasses in prominent places to ensure that it is always available. It is more convenient to drink consistently when there is water readily available.

Drink with Meals: To promote healthy digestion and sufficient hydration, have a glass of water with every meal. Water consumption with meals can also increase feelings of fullness and satisfaction, which may lessen the need to snack in between meals.

Water is the Best Drink to Start and End the Day: Have a glass of water as soon as you get up and one more glass right before bed. This makes sure you're properly hydrated before bed and helps you start drinking more water in the morning.

You may boost your water intake and take advantage of the many health advantages of staying hydrated by implementing these techniques into your everyday routine. Always pay attention to your body's thirst signals and modify your water consumption as necessary, particularly in hot weather or at times when you're exercising more.

Observations and Warnings

There are a few things to bear in mind and cautions to be aware of while deciding if drinking more water can aid in weight loss:

Not a Magic Bullet: Although drinking more water is good for your general health and wellbeing, it won't likely result in noticeable weight loss on its own. Water consumption is only one component of a comprehensive weight-management strategy that also consists of behavior modification techniques, a balanced diet, and regular exercise.

Caloric Content: While water has no calories by itself, other drinks like sugar-filled sodas, juices, and sports drinks can add a lot of calories to your diet. Water can help you cut calories overall and aid in weight loss by substituting high-calorie drinks with less.

Appetite Regulation: Having a glass of water prior to eating may assist increase feelings of fullness and curb appetite, which will result in consuming fewer calories throughout meals. Individual differences may exist in the impact on appetite suppression, and in certain situations, consuming water may not be enough to regulate hunger.

Metabolic Rate: According to certain research, consuming cold water may momentarily raise metabolic rate, which would result in higher calorie expenditure. But the benefit is just temporary, and drinking water by itself isn't likely to speed up metabolism sufficiently to result in noticeable weight reduction.

Individual Variability: Different people will experience different effects from drinking water when it comes to losing weight. Drinking more water may have different effects on weight control depending on a number of factors, including age, gender, weight, exercise level, and general food quality.

Water Retention: Intriguingly, the body's defense mechanism of holding onto water can cause dehydration to cause water retention. Therefore, although more water consumption may not always result in greater fluid loss, remaining well hydrated is crucial for reducing water retention and maintaining fluid balance.

Status of Your Hydration: To stay properly hydrated, pay attention to your body's thirst signals and sip water when you feel it. But, you shouldn't push yourself to consume more water than your body needs because doing so could put your health at danger for electrolyte imbalances, overhydration, and other problems.

Underlying Health Conditions: A number of illnesses, including heart failure, renal disease, and electrolyte imbalances, can alter fluid balance and necessitate close monitoring of fluid intake. A healthcare provider should be consulted by those who have these problems before making big adjustments to their water intake.

Although drinking water to stay hydrated is beneficial to general health and may support weight loss attempts by lowering caloric intake and increasing feelings of fullness, it is only one part of an all-encompassing weight management strategy. In order to reach and stay at a healthy weight, it's critical to have a holistic approach to weight loss and take into account a variety of aspects, such as diet, physical activity, and personal lifestyle choices. Speaking with a registered dietician or other healthcare expert can help you receive individualized advice and support that is catered to your requirements and objectives.

Summary

In conclusion, there is a complicated and nuanced relationship between increasing water consumption and weight loss. Even though drinking more water can help with weight management in some ways, such boosting feelings of fullness, cutting calories, and enhancing general hydration, it is not a miracle weight-loss tactic.

While maintaining enough water is crucial for general health and wellbeing, especially while trying to lose weight, it's also critical to treat hydration as one component of a holistic plan that also involves behavior adjustment, regular exercise, and a balanced diet.

While switching to water from sugary drinks might reduce overall calorie consumption and help suppress desire and reduce calorie intake, other important factors that affect weight control include individual metabolism, dietary habits, and lifestyle choices.

In the end, even while increasing your water intake can help you live a healthier lifestyle and lose weight, it's crucial to set reasonable goals and concentrate on creating long-lasting dietary and lifestyle adjustments for long-term success. A licensed dietician or other healthcare expert can offer individualized advice and support to help people reach their weight loss objectives in a safe and efficient manner.

THE END